Soup Cookbook
Fast and Easy Gluten Free Soup Recipes
Inspired by the Mediterranean Diet

MW01295425

by Vesela Tabakova
Text copyright(c)2016 Vesela Tabakova

Table Of Contents

Rapid Weight Loss Soups the Whole Family Will Love

Following a gluten-free diet is extremely challenging and often very expensive. Gluten-free foods are hard to find, do not always taste very good and many people who have to avoid gluten feel overwhelmed and depressed by the fact that they have to follow this diet.

The truth is, however, that there is an easy and simple way to stick to a gluten-free diet by focusing on naturally gluten-free whole foods. So much of the food you already love is naturally gluten-free and, therefore, the safest and most nutritious way to follow a gluten-free diet is to cook at home and to stick primarily to fresh, unrefined and unprocessed ingredients. If you want to eat really healthy food with good ingredients, it is best to make it yourself. It's really not that difficult to prepare your meals at home with fresh vegetables, herbs, meat, rice and beans, as well as other naturally gluten-free foods such as quinoa or buckwheat.

Planning simple, home cooked meals and choosing naturally gluten-free whole foods should make your transition to a gluten-free lifestyle much easier. Here are some easy-to-make homemade gluten-free soup recipes to get you cooking.

Turkey and Quinoa Meatball Soup

Serves 5-6

Ingredients:

1 lb ground turkey

1 large egg

2 tbsp fresh parsley, finely chopped

1 medium onion, grated

salt and black pepper, to taste

5 cups gluten-free vegetable broth

1 medium carrot, chopped

1 onion, chopped

2 garlic cloves, chopped

1 green pepper, chopped

1 potato, peeled and cubed

1/3 cup quinoa, washed

salt and black pepper, to taste

Directions:

Combine the onion, egg, fresh parsley, salt and pepper in a large bowl and stir. Add in the ground turkey and mix with hands. Roll tablespoonfuls of the mixture into balls. Place on a large plate or baking sheet until ready to cook.

In a large saucepan over medium heat, heat the olive oil. Add in carrot, onion and garlic and cook, stirring, for about 1-2 minutes. Add vegetable broth and bring to the boil.

Add meatballs, potato, pepper and quinoa and simmer, uncovered, about 15 minutes. Season with salt and pepper. Serve with lemon juice.

Chicken and Buckwheat Soup

Serves 6-7

Ingredients:

2 lb chicken breasts

2-3 carrots, chopped

1 celery rib, chopped

1 onion, chopped

8 cups water

1/3 cup buckwheat groats

1/2 tsp salt

ground black pepper, to taste

lemon juice, to serve

fresh parsley, to serve

Directions:

Place chicken breasts in a soup pot. Add onion, carrots, celery, salt, pepper and water. Stir well and bring to a boil. Add buckwheat, stir, and reduce heat. Simmer for 30 minutes.

Remove chicken from pot and let it cool slightly. Shred it and return it to pot. Serve soup with lemon juice and sprinkled with fresh parsley.

Greek Lemon Chicken Soup

Serves 4

Ingredients:

2 lb chicken breast, diced

1/3 cup rice

2 cups gluten-free chicken broth

3 cups water

1 onion, finely cut

2 raw eggs

3 tbsp olive oil

1/2 cup fresh lemon juice

1 tbsp salt

1 tsp ground pepper

a bunch of fresh parsley for garnish, finely cut

Directions:

In a medium pot, heat the olive oil and sauté the onions until they are soft and translucent. Add the chicken broth and water together with the washed rice and bring everything to a boil. Reduce heat and simmer. When the rice is almost done, add the diced chicken breast to the pot. Let it cook for another five minutes, or until the chicken is cooked through.

Beat the eggs and lemon juice together in a separate bowl. Pour two cups of broth slowly into the egg mixture, whisking constantly. When all the broth is incorporated, add this mixture to the chicken soup and stir well to blend. Do not boil any more. Season with salt and pepper and garnish with parsley. Serve hot.

Lemon Chicken and Kale Soup

Serves 5-6

Ingredients:

1 cup cooked chicken, cubed or shredded

1 small onion, chopped

1 small carrot, grated

1 bunch kale, cut into 1 inch pieces

4 cups chicken broth

1 tsp Worcestershire sauce

1 tsp Dijon mustard

3 tbsp olive oil

1 tsp paprika

3 tbsp lemon juice

1 tsp grated lemon zest

salt and black pepper, to taste

grated Parmezan cheese, to serve

Directions:

Heat a soup pot over medium heat. Gently sauté onion, garlic and carrot, stirring occasionally. Stir in the lemon zest, chicken broth, Worcestershire sauce, Dijon mustard and cooked chicken.

Bring to a boil then reduce heat and simmer for 10 minutes. Stir in the kale and simmer for 3-4 minutes or until kale is tender.

Stir in the lemon juice and season with salt and pepper to taste. Serve sprinkled with Parmezan cheese.

Slow Cooker French-style Farmhouse Chicken Soup

Serves 5-6

Ingredients:

4 skinless, boneless chicken thighs, cut into bite-sized pieces

1 leek, trimmed, halved, finely cut

1 celery rib, trimmed, halved, finely cut

2 carrots, chopped

1 fennel bulb, trimmed, diced

1 cup frozen peas

4 cups chicken broth

1 tsp thyme

1 tsp salt

Directions:

Combine all ingredients in the slow cooker. Cover and cook on low for 6-7 hours.

Chicken Vegetable Soup

Serves 6-7

Ingredients:

2 lb boneless chicken thighs, cut in bite sized pieces

1 small onion, chopped

1 celery rib, chopped

1/2 small parsnip, chopped

3 garlic cloves, chopped

1 carrot, chopped

1 red bell pepper, chopped

1 lb potatoes, peeled and cubed

5 cups chicken broth

1 tsp thyme

2 bay leaves

1 tsp salt

black pepper, to taste

1 tsp summer savory

Directions:

Season the chicken well with salt, ground black pepper and summer savory. Place it in a slow cooker with all remaining ingredients.

Cover and cook on low for 6-7 hours or on high for 4 hours.

Moroccan Chicken and Butternut Squash Soup

Serves 6-7

Ingredients:

3 skinless, boneless chicken thighs, cut into bite-sized pieces

1 big onion, chopped

1 zucchini, quartered lengthwise and sliced into 1/2-inch pieces

3 cups peeled butternut squash, cut in 1/2-inch pieces

2 tbsp tomato paste

5 cups gluten-free chicken broth

1/2 tsp ground cumin

1/4 tsp ground cinnamon

1 tsp paprika

1 tsp salt

2 tbsp fresh basil leaves, chopped

1 tbsp grated orange rind

3 tbsp olive oil

Directions:

Heat a soup pot over medium heat. Gently sauté onion, for 3-4 minutes, stirring occasionally. Add chicken pieces and cook for 4 minutes, until chicken is brown on all sides. Add cumin, cinnamon and paprika and stir well. Add butternut squash and tomato paste; stir again. Add chicken broth and bring to a boil, then reduce heat and simmer 10 minutes. Stir in salt and zucchini pieces; cook until squash is tender.

Remove pot from heat. Season with salt and pepper to taste. Stir in chopped basil and orange rind and serve.

Balkan Chicken Soup

Serves 6-7

Ingredients:

1 whole chicken (3-4 lbs), cut into sections

5 cups water

1 large onion, whole

1 large onion, chopped

3 garlic cloves, chopped

2 carrots, chopped

1 red bell pepper

1 tsp savory

1 tsp thyme

2 bay leaves

2 tbsp olive oil

1 tsp salt

black pepper, to taste

Directions:

Place the chicken, bay leaves, salt, whole onion and whole red pepper into a pot with five cups of cold water. Bring the pot to boil, reduce heat and simmer for one hour, scooping out any solid foam that settles at the top. When ready, strain the broth and reserve.

Remove the meat from the chicken and cut into large chunks. Discard the bay leaves, the onion and the pepper. Place the pot back on the stove, heat the olive oil and sauté the chopped onion, garlic, carrots and thyme for about 5 minutes. Pour in the broth and season with salt and pepper. Simmer for about 15 minutes or until the vegetables are tender. Add in the chicken pieces and the savory. Simmer for 10 more minutes and serve warm.

Brown Lentil and Beef Soup

Serves 6

Ingredients:

1 lb ground beef

1 cup brown lentils

2 carrots, chopped

1 large onion, chopped

1 potato, cut into 1/2 inch cubes

4 garlic cloves, chopped

2 tomatoes, grated or pureed

5 cups water

1 tsp savory

1 tsp oregano

1 tsp paprika

2 tbsp olive oil

1 tsp salt

ground black pepper, to taste

Directions:

Heat olive oil in a large soup pot. Brown beef, breaking it up with a spoon. Add paprika and garlic and stir. Add lentils, remaining vegetables, water and spice.

Bring to a boil. Reduce heat to low and simmer, covered, for about an hour, or until lentils are tender. Stir occasionally.

Beef and Vegetable Soup

Serves 6-8

Ingredients:

2 lbs stewing beef

3 tbsp olive oil

1 large onion, chopped

1 cup mushrooms, chopped

2 carrots, chopped

1 celery rib, chopped

6 cups water

2 tbsp tomato paste

1/2 cup parsley, chopped

salt and black pepper, to taste

Directions:

Season the beef pieces with salt and pepper. In a large soup pot, heat olive oil and seal the beef in batches then set it aside in a plate, covered. Sauté the onions, mushrooms, carrots, and celery over medium high heat.

Return the meat to the pot, add water and bring to the boil. Reduce heat and simmer, covered, for about an hour, stirring occasionally. Dissolve the tomato paste in a few tablespoons of the soup broth and add it to the pot. Stir in the chopped parsley and season with salt and pepper to taste.

Beef and Vegetable Minestrone

Serves 5-6

Ingredients:

2 slices bacon, chopped

1 cup ground beef

2 carrots, chopped

2 cloves garlic, finely chopped

1 large onion, chopped

1 celery rib, chopped

1 bay leaf

1 tsp dried basil

1 tsp dried rosemary, crushed

1/4 tsp crushed chillies

1 can tomatoes, chopped

5 cups gluten-free beef broth

Directions:

In a large saucepan, cook bacon and ground beef until well done, breaking up the beef as it cooks. Drain off the fat and add carrots, garlic, onion and celery.

Cook, stirring, for about 5 minutes or until the onions are translucent. Season with the bay leaf, basil, rosemary and crushed chillies. Stir in tomatoes and beef broth. Bring to a boil then reduce heat and simmer for about 30 minutes.

Italian Meatball Soup

Serves 4-5

Ingredients:

1 lb lean ground beef

1 small onion, grated

1 onion, chopped

2 garlic cloves, crushed

1 zucchini, diced

3-4 basil leaves, finely chopped

1 egg, lightly beaten

2 cups gluten-free tomato sauce with basil

3 cups water

2 tbsp olive oil

salt and black pepper, to taste

Directions:

Combine ground beef, grated onion, garlic, basil and egg in a large bowl. Season with salt and pepper. Mix well with hands and roll tablespoonfuls of the mixture into balls. Place on a large plate.

Heat olive oil into a large deep saucepan and sauté onion and garlic until transparent. Add tomato sauce, water, and bring to the boil over high heat. Add in the meatballs. Reduce heat to medium-low and simmer, uncovered, for 10 minutes.

Meatball Soup

Serves 4-5

Ingredients:

1 lb lean ground beef

1 onion, chopped

2 garlic cloves, cut

1 tomato, diced

1 carrot, diced

1 potato, cubed

1 green pepper, chopped

3 cups water

½ bunch of parsley, finely cut

3 tbsp olive oil

½ tsp black pepper

1 tsp savory

1 tsp paprika

1 tsp salt

Directions:

Combine ground meat, savory, paprika, black pepper and salt in a large bowl. Mix well with hands and roll teaspoonfuls of the mixture into balls. Heat olive oil into a large soup pot and sauté onion and garlic until transparent.

Add in water and bring to the boil over high heat. Add the meatballs, carrot, potato and green pepper. Reduce heat to low and simmer, uncovered, for 15 minutes. Add the tomato and the parsley and cook for 5 more minutes.

Lamb Soup

Serves 4-5

Ingredients:

2 lb lean boneless lamb, cubed

1 onion, finely cut

1 carrot, chopped

4-5 spring onions, chopped

1/3 cup rice, washed and drained

1 tomato, diced

4 cups hot water

2 tbsp sunflower oil

1 tsp salt

black pepper, to taste

1 tbsp dry mint

1/2 cup parsley, finely cut

3 tbsp yogurt

1 egg

Directions:

Heat 2 tablespoonfuls of sunflower oil and gently brown the lamb cubes in a medium sized cooking pot. Add the finely cut onion and the carrot and saute for a minute or two, stirring. Add two cups of hot water and bring to the boil, then lower heat to medium-low and simmer until the lamb softens. Add in 2 more cups of hot water, rice, butter, green onions, tomato, mint, salt and black pepper. Bring to a boil again and simmer until the rice is done.

Whisk the the egg and the yogurt in a small bowl. Take one ladle from the soup and add into the egg mixture, whisk. Take another and whisk again. Pour this mixture back into into the soup and stir. Do not boil. Sprinkle with parsley and serve while still hot.

Buckwheat Fish Soup

Serves 4

Ingredients:

2 lb fish steaks, cut into 1 inch pieces

4 cups water

1/3 cup buckwheat, washed

2 medium potatoes, diced

2 carrots, grated

1 medium onion, chopped

1 bay leave

1/2 cup fresh dill, chopped

lemon juice, to serve

salt and black pepper, to taste

Directions:

Place the fish, bay leave, vegetables and buckwheat groats in a pot with four cups of cold water. Bring the pot to a boil then lower heat. Simmer until fish and potatoes are done. Season with dill, salt and black pepper just before serving. Serve with lemon juice

Spanish Seafood Soup

Serves 4-5

Ingredients:

2 lbs whole raw prawns

1 lb mussels

4 cups cold water

3 spring onions, chopped

1 bell pepper, finely chopped

2 large tomatoes, diced

1 tbsp tomato puree

2 garlic cloves, minced

2 tbsp olive oil

2 bay leaves

1 tsp paprika

½ tsp cayenne pepper

salt and pepper, to taste

the juice of one small lemon

a bunch of parsley, chopped

Directions:

De-head and de-shell the prawns and leave them in a bowl to the side. Put the heads and shells in a pan with cold water. Add the bay leaves, bring to the boil and reduce heat.

Simmer for 20 minutes. While the broth is simmering, sauté the shallots and pepper in olive oil for 5 minutes, then add the garlic for two more minutes.

When the broth is ready strain it and add it to the the shallots. Bring to the boil, add the tomatoes and tomato puree, the prawns, the mussels and simmer for 10 more minutes. In the end add the paprika and cayenne pepper, season to taste with salt and pepper and add the lemon juice. Garnish with parsley and serve.

Hot Spanish Squid Soup

Serves 4

Ingredients:

1 lb Squid; cleaned, cut into 1 inch pieces

2 garlic cloves; crushed

1/2 cup tomato puree or chopped tomatoes

3 cups water

1 tbsp olive oil

black pepper, to taste

1/2 cup parsley, finely chopped, to serve

Directions:

Heat olive oil in a soup pot over medium high heat and gently sauté garlic just for a minute. Add squid and sauté for 2-3 minutes, stirring. Add black pepper, tomato sauce or tomatoes and water. Bring to a boil and let simmer soup for an hour. Serve sprinkled with parsley.

Chilled Celery and Prawn Soup

Serves 4-5

Ingredients:

12 cooked prawns, peeled and coarsely chopped

4 celery ribs, trimmed and chopped

2 leeks, only pale section, chopped

2 potatoes, diced

4 cups gluten-free chicken broth

1 cup coconut milk

3 tbsp sunflower oil

a pinch of cayenne pepper

1 tsp chopped fresh tarragon

Directions:

Heat the sunflower oil in a medium saucepan over medium heat. Sauté the celery and leeks, stirring, for 3-4 minutes or until the leeks are soft.

Add in the potatoes, chicken broth, milk, cayenne pepper and the tarragon. Simmer for about 30 minutes, stirring occasionally, until the potatoes are done. Set aside for 5 minutes to cool slightly.

Blend until smooth and place in the fridge until well chilled. Serve topped with the prawns.

Dump Bean and Bacon Soup

Serves 5-6

Ingredients:

1 slices bacon, chopped

1 can Black Beans, rinsed

1 can Kidney Beans, rinsed

1 celery rib, chopped

1/2 red onion, chopped

1 can tomatoes, diced, undrained

4 cups water

1 tsp smoked paprika

1 tsp dried mint

1/2 cup fresh parsley

ground black pepper, to taste

Directions:

Dump all ingredients in a soup pot. Stir well and bring to a boil. Reduce heat and simmer for 35 minutes.

Season with salt and black pepper to taste, and serve.

Lemon Artichoke Soup

Serves 4-5

Ingredients:

2 cups artichoke hearts, chopped

1 small onion, very finely cut

1 celery rib, very finely cut

2 carrots, very finely cut

1 garlic clove, crushed

3 cups gluten-free chicken broth

2 tbsp olive oil

1 tsp salt

1 tsp black pepper

1 fresh lemon, halved

2 cups coconut milk

Directions:

Heat olive oil in a large pot and gently sauté onion, celery, carrot and garlic. Stir in chicken broth, artichokes, salt and pepper and bring to the boil. Lower heat and simmer for 10 minutes.

Remove from heat and blend until smooth. Return to heat, juice half a lemon into soup. Bring to the boil, reduce heat and simmer for 5 more minutes. Stir in coconut milk and simmer for another 5 minutes.

Beetroot and Carrot Soup

Serves 6

Ingredients:

4 beets, washed and peeled

2 carrots, peeled, chopped

2 potatoes, peeled, chopped

1 medium onion, chopped

2 cups gluten-free vegetable broth

2 cups water

2 tbsp yogurt

2 tbsp olive oil

a bunch or spring onions, chopped, to serve

Directions:

Peel and chop the beets. Heat olive oil in a saucepan over medium high heat and sauté the onion and carrot until onion is tender. Add beets, potatoes, broth and water. Bring to the boil. Reduce heat to medium and simmer, partially covered, for 30-40 minutes, or until beets are tender. Cool slightly.

Blend soup in batches until smooth. Return it to pan over low heat and cook, stirring, for 4 to 5 minutes or until heated through. Season with salt and pepper. Serve soup topped with yogurt and sprinkled with spring onions.

Minted Pea Soup

Serves 4

Ingredients:

1 onion, finely chopped

2 garlic cloves, finely chopped

3 cups gluten-free vegetable broth

1/3 cup mint leaves

2 lb green peas, frozen

3 tbsp olive oil

1/4 cup yogurt, to serve

small mint leaves, to serve

Directions:

Heat oil in a large saucepan over medium-high heat and sauté onion and garlic for 5 minutes or until soft.

Add gluten-free vegetable broth and bring to the boil, then add mint and peas. Cover, reduce heat, and cook for 3 minutes, or until peas are tender but still green. Remove from heat. Set aside to cool slightly, then blend in batches, until smooth. Return soup to saucepan over medium-low heat and cook until heated through. Season with salt and pepper. Serve topped with yogurt, black pepper and mint leaves.

White Bean Soup

Serves 6

Ingredients:

1 cup white beans

2-3 carrots

2 onions, finely chopped

1-2 tomatoes, grated

1 red bell pepper, chopped

4-5 springs of fresh mint and parsley

1 tsp paprika

3 tbsp sunflower oil

salt, to taste

Directions:

Soak the beans in cold water for 3-4 hours, drain and discard the water. Cover the beans with cold water. Add the oil, finely chopped carrots, onions and pepper.

Bring to the boil and simmer until the beans are tender. Add the grated tomatoes, mint, paprika and salt. Simmer for another 15 minutes. Serve sprinkled with finely chopped parsley.

Brown Lentil Soup

Serves 6-7

Ingredients:

2 cups brown lentils

2 onions, chopped

5-6 cloves garlic, peeled

3 medium carrots, chopped

2-3 medium tomatoes, ripe

4-5 cups of water

4 tbsp olive oil

1 ½ tsp paprika

1 tbsp savory

Directions:

Heat the oil in a cooking pot, add the onions and carrots and sauté until golden. Add the paprika and washed lentils with 3-4 cups of warm water; continue to simmer.

Chop the tomatoes and add them to the soup, about 15 min after the lentils have started to simmer. Add savory and peeled garlic cloves. Let the soup simmer until the lentils are soft. Salt to taste.

Moroccan Lentil Soup

Serves 6-7

Ingredients:

1 cup red lentils

1 cup canned chickpeas, drained

2 onions, chopped

2 cloves garlic, minced

1 cup canned tomatoes, chopped

1 cup canned white beans, drained

3 carrots, diced

3 celery ribs, diced

5 cups water

1 tsp ginger, grated

1 tsp ground cardamom

½ tsp ground cumin

3 tbsp olive oil

Directions:

In a large pot, sauté onions, garlic and ginger in olive oil, for about 5 minutes. Add the water, lentils, chickpeas, white beans, tomatoes, carrots, celery, cardamom and cumin.

Bring to a boil for a few minutes, then simmer for ½ hour or longer, until the lentils are tender. Puree half the soup in a food processor or blender. Return the pureed soup to the pot, stir and serve.

Pumpkin and Bell Pepper Soup

Serves 4

Ingredients:

1 medium leek, chopped

9 oz pumpkin, peeled, deseeded, cut into small cubes

1/2 red bell pepper, cut into small pieces

1 can tomatoes, undrained, crushed

3 cups gluten-free vegetable broth

1/2 tsp ground cumin

salt and black pepper, to taste

Directions:

Heat the olive oil in a medium saucepan and sauté the leek for 4-5 minutes. Add the pumpkin and bell pepper and cook, stirring, for 2-3 minutes. Add tomatoes, broth and cumin and bring to the boil.

Cover, reduce heat to low and simmer, stirring occasionally, for 30 minutes or until vegetables are soft. Season with salt and pepper and leave aside to cool. Blend in batches and re-heat to serve.

Spicy Carrot Soup

Serves 6-8

Ingredients:

10 carrots, peeled and chopped

2 medium onions, chopped

4-5 cups water

5 tbsp coconut oil

2 cloves garlic, minced

1 red chili pepper, finely chopped

1/2 bunch, fresh coriander, finely cut

salt and pepper to taste

Directions:

Heat the coconut oil in a large pot over medium heat, and sauté the onions, carrots, garlic and chili pepper until tender. Add 4-5 cups of water and bring to a boil. Reduce heat to low and simmer 30 minutes.

Transfer the soup to a blender or food processor and blend until smooth. Return to the pot, and continue cooking for a few more minutes. Remove soup from heat, and set aside for a few minutes. Serve with coriander sprinkled over each serving.

Mushroom Soup

Serves 4

Ingredients:

2 cups mushrooms, peeled and chopped

1 onion, chopped

2 cloves of garlic, crushed and chopped

1 tsp dried thyme

3 cups gluten-free vegetable broth

salt and pepper, to taste

3 tbsp coconut or olive oil

Directions:

Sauté onions and garlic in a large soup pot untill transparent. Add in thyme and the mushrooms.

Cook, stirring, for 10 minutes then add vegetable broth and simmer for another 10-20 minutes. Blend, season and serve.

Tomato and Quinoa Soup

Serves 4-5

Ingredients:

4 cups chopped fresh tomatoes or 2 cups canned tomatoes

1 large onion, diced

1/3 cup quinoa, washed very well

3 cups water

4 garlic cloves, minced

3 tbsp olive oil

1 tsp salt

½ tsp black pepper

1 tsp sugar

½ bunch of fresh parsley

Directions:

Sauté onions and garlic in oil in a large soup pot. When onions have softened, add tomatoes and cook until onions are golden and tomatoes soft. Stir in the spices and mix well to coat vegetables.

Blend the soup then return to the pot. Add the water, quinoa and a teaspoon of sugar and bring to a boil, then reduce heat and simmer 20 minutes stirring occasionally. Sprinkle with parsley and serve.

Spinach, Leek and Quinoa Soup

Serves 6

Ingredients:

½ cup quinoa

2 leeks halved lengthwise and sliced

1 onion, chopped

2 garlic cloves, chopped

1 tbsp olive oil

1 can of diced tomatoes, undrained

2 cups of fresh spinach, cut

4-5 cups gluten-free vegetable broth

salt and pepper, to taste

Directions:

Heat olive oil in a large pot over medium heat and sauté onion for 2 minutes. Add in the leeks and cook for another 2-3 minutes, then add garlic and stir.

Season with salt and pepper to taste. Add the vegetable broth, canned tomatoes and quinoa. Bring to a boil then reduce heat and simmer for 10 minutes. Stir in the spinach and cook for another 5 minutes.

Vegetable Quinoa Soup

Serves 6

Ingredients:

½ cup quinoa

1 onion, chopped

1 potato, diced

1 carrot, diced

1 red bell pepper, chopped

2 tomatoes, chopped

1 zucchini, diced

1 teaspoon dried oregano

3-4 tbsp olive oil

black pepper, to taste

5 cups water

2 tbsp fresh lemon juice

Directions:

Rinse quinoa very well in a fine mesh strainer under running water; set aside to drain.

Heat the oil in a large soup pot and gently sauté the onions and carrot for 2-3 minutes, stirring every now and then. Add in the potato, bell pepper, tomatoes, spices and water. Stir to combine.

Cover, bring to a boil, then lower heat and simmer for 10 minutes. Add in the quinoa and the zucchini; cover and simmer for 15 minutes or until the vegetables are tender. Add in the lemon juice; stir to combine.

Spinach and Mushrooms Soup

Serves 4-5

Ingredients:

1 small onion, finely cut

1 small carrot, chopped

1 small zucchini, diced

2 medium potatoes, diced

5-6 white mushrooms, chopped

2 cups chopped fresh spinach

3 cups gluten-free vegetable broth

4 tbsp olive oil

salt and black pepper to taste

Directions:

Heat olive oil in a large pot over medium heat. Add potatoes, onions and mushroom and cook until vegetables are soft but not mushy.

Add chopped fresh spinach, zucchini, vegetable broth and simmer for about 20 minutes. Season to taste with salt and pepper.

Broccoli and Potato Soup

Serves 6

Ingredients:

2 lbs broccoli, cut into florets

2 potatoes, chopped

1 big onion, chopped

3 garlic cloves, crushed

4 cups water

1 tbsp olive oil

¼ tsp ground nutmeg

Directions:

Heat oil in a large saucepan over medium-high heat. Add onion and garlic and sauté, stirring, for 3 minutes or until soft.

Add broccoli, potato and 4 cups of cold water. Cover and bring to the boil, then reduce heat to low. Simmer, stirring, for 10 to 15 minutes, or until potato is tender. Remove from heat. Blend until smooth. Return to pan. Cook for 5 minutes or until heated through. Season with nutmeg and pepper before serving.

Creamy Potato Soup

Serves 5-6

Ingredients:

4-5 medium potatoes, cut into small cubes

2 carrots, chopped

1 zucchini, chopped

1 celery rib, chopped

3 cups water

3 tbsp olive oil

1 cup whole milk

½ tsp dried rosemary

salt to taste

black pepper to taste

a bunch of fresh parsley for garnish, finely cut

Directions:

Heat the olive oil over medium heat and sauté the vegetables for 2-3 minutes. Pour 3 cups of water, add the rosemary and bring the soup to a boil, then lower heat and simmer until all the vegetables are tender.

Blend soup in a blender until smooth. Add a cup of warm milk and blend some more. Serve warm, seasoned with black pepper and parsley sprinkled over each serving.

Leek, Rice and Potato Soup

Serves 6

Ingredients:

2-3 potatoes, diced

1 small onion, chopped

1 leek halved lengthwise and sliced

1/3 cup rice

4-5 cups of water

3 tbsp olive oil

lemon juice, to serve

Directions:

Heat a soup pot over medium heat. Add olive oil and sauté onion for 2 minutes. Add leeks and potatoes and cook for a few minutes more.

Add three cups of water, bring the soup to a boil then reduce heat and simmer for 5 minutes. Add the very well washed rice and simmer for 10 more minutes. Serve with lemon juice to taste.

Bulgarian Potato Soup

Serves 4-5

Ingredients:

1 medium onion, chopped

4-5 medium potatoes, diced

3 cups water

3 tbsp sunflower oil

1 1/2 cup whole milk

1 tsp paprika

salt to taste

black pepper, to taste

Directions:

Heat the sunflower oil over medium heat and sauté the onion for 2-3 minutes. Add the diced potatoes and stir. Add a teaspoon of paprika and stir again.

Pour 2 cups of water and bring the soup to a boil, then lower heat and simmer until the potatoes are tender. Stir in the milk, season with salt and pepper to taste and simmer for 1-2 minutes. Serve with lemon juice to taste

Shredded Cabbage Soup

Serves 4

Ingredients:

1 large onion, finely chopped

3 tbsp sunflower oil

3 cups gluten-free beef broth

1 small cabbage, shredded

1 carrot, sliced

1 medium potato, diced

1 celery rib, sliced

2 tomatoes, diced

1/2 tsp cumin

salt, to taste

black pepper, to taste

Directions:

Heat the sunflower oil over medium heat and gently sauté the onion for 2-3 minutes. Add cabbage and stir; add in carrots, potatoes, celery, tomatoes and cummin and stir again.

Add in in the beef broth and enough water to thoroughly cover all ingredients. Bring the soup to a boil, reduce heat and simmer for 1 hour. Season with salt and black pepper to taste.

Mediterranean Chickpea Soup

Serves 5-6

Ingredients:

2 cups canned chickpeas, drained

a bunch of green onions, finely cut

2 cloves garlic, crushed

1 cup canned tomatoes, diced

5 cups gluten-free vegetable broth

3 tbsp olive oil

1 bay leaf

½ tsp crushed rosemary

½ cup freshly grated Parmesan cheese

Directions:

Sauté onion and garlic in olive oil in a heavy soup pot. Add broth, chickpeas, tomato, bay leaf, and rosemary.

Bring to the boil, then reduce heath and simmer for 20 minutes. Remove from heat and serve sprinkled with Parmesan cheese.

Carrot and Chickpea Soup

Serves 4-5

Ingredients:

3-4 big carrots, chopped

1 leek, chopped

4 cups gluten-free vegetable broth

1 cup canned chickpeas, undrained

½ cup orange juice

2 tbsp olive oil

½ tsp cumin

½ tsp ginger

4-5 tbsp yogurt, to serve

Directions:

Heat oil in a large saucepan over medium heat. Add leek and carrots and sauté until soft. Add in orange juice, broth, chickpeas and spices.

Bring to the boil then reduce heat to medium-low and simmer, covered, for 15 minutes. Blend soup until smooth; return to pan. Season with salt and pepper. Stir over heat until heated through. Pour in 4-5 bowls, top with yogurt and serve.

Roasted Red Pepper Soup

Serves 6-7

Ingredients:

5-6 red peppers

1 large onion, chopped

2 garlic cloves, crushed

4 medium tomatoes, chopped

4 cups gluten-free vegetable broth

3 tbsp olive oil

2 bay leaves

Directions:

Grill the peppers or roast them in the oven at 480 F until the skins are a little burnt. Place the roasted peppers in a brown paper bag or a lidded container and leave covered for about 10 minutes. This makes it easier to peel them. Peel the skins and remove the seeds. Cut the peppers in small pieces.

Heat oil in a large saucepan over medium-high heat. Add onion and garlic and sauté, stirring, for 3 minutes or until onion has softened. Add the red peppers, bay leaves, tomato and simmer for 5 minutes.

Add broth. Season with pepper. Bring to the boil then reduce heat and simmer for 20 minutes. Set aside to cool slightly. Blend, in batches, until smooth and serve.

Spring Nettle Soup

Serves 6

Ingredients:

1.5 lb young top shoots of nettles, well washed

1 cup spinach leaves

1 carrot, chopped

a bunch of spring onions, coarsely chopped

3 tbsp sunflower oil

3 cups hot water

1 tsp salt

Directions:

Clean the young nettles, wash and cook them in slightly salted water. Drain, rinse, drain again and then chop or pass through a sieve. Sauté the chopped spring onions and carrot in the oil until the onion softens.

Add in the nettles and spinach leaves and gradually stir in the water. Bring to a boil, reduce heat and simmer for 5 minutes. Set aside to cool then blend in batches. Serve with a dollop of yogurt.

Gazpacho

Serves 6-7

Ingredients:

6-7 medium tomatoes, peeled and halved

1 onion, sliced

1 green pepper, sliced

1 big cucumber, peeled and sliced

2 cloves garlic

salt, to taste

4 tbsp olive oil

to garnish

1/2 onion, chopped

1 green pepper, chopped

1 cucumber, chopped

Directions:

Place the tomatoes, garlic, onion, green pepper, cucumber, salt and olive oil in a blender or food processor and puree until smooth, adding small amounts of cold water if needed to achieve desired consistency. Serve the gazpacho chilled with the chopped onion, green pepper and cucumber.

Avocado Gazpacho

Serves 4

Ingredients:

2 ripe avocados, peeled, pitted and diced

1 cup tomatoes, diced

1 cup cucumbers, peeled and diced

1 small onion, chopped

2 tbsp lemon juice

1 tsp salt

black pepper, to taste

Directions:

Place avocados, cucumbers, tomatoes, onion, lemon juice and salt and pepper in a blender. Blend until smooth and serve sprinkled with cilantro or parsley leaves.

Cold Cucumber Soup

Serves 4-5

Ingredients:

1 large or two small cucumbers

2 cups yogurt

2-3 cloves garlic, crushed or chopped

1 cup cold water

4 tbsp sunflower or olive oil

2 bunches of fresh dill, finely chopped

1/2 cup crushed walnuts

Directions:

Wash the cucumber, peel and cut it into small cubes. In a large bowl dilute the yogurt with water to taste, add the cucumber and garlic stirring well. Add salt to the taste, garnish with the dill and the crushed walnuts and put in the fridge to cool.

FREE BONUS RECIPES: 20 Superfood Paleo and Vegan Smoothies for Vibrant Health and Easy Weight Loss

Winter Greens Smoothie

Serves: 2

Prep time: 5 min

Ingredients:

2 broccoli florets, frozen

1½ cup coconut water

½ banana

½ cup pineapple

1 cup fresh spinach

2 kale leaves

Directions:

Combine ingredients in blender and blend until smooth. Enjoy!

Delicious Kale Smoothie

Serves: 2

Prep time: 5 min

Ingredients:

2-3 ice cubes

1½ cup apple juice

3-4 kale leaves

1 apple, cut

1 cup strawberries

½ tsp cloves

Directions:

Combine ingredients in blender and purée until smooth.

Cherry Smoothie

Serves: 2

Prep time: 5 min

Ingredients:

2-3 ice cubes

1½ cup almond or coconut milk

1½ cup pitted and frozen cherries

½ avocado

1 tsp cinnamon

1 tsp chia seeds

Directions :

Combine all ingredients into a blender and process until smooth. Enjoy!

Banana and Coconut Smoothie

Serves: 2

Prep time: 5 min

Ingredients:

1 frozen banana, chopped

1½ cup coconut water

2-3 small broccoli florets

1 tbsp coconut butter

Directions :

Add all ingredients into a blender and blend until the smoothie turns into an even and smooth consistency. Enjoy!

Avocado and Pineapple Smoothie

Serves: 2

Prep time: 5 min

Ingredients:

3-4 ice cubes

1½ cup coconut water

½ avocado

2 cups diced pineapple

Directions:

Combine all ingredients in a blender, and blend until smooth. Enjoy!

Carrot and Mango Smoothie

Serves: 2

Prep time: 5 min

Ingredients:

1 cup frozen mango chunks

1 cup carrot juice

½ cup orange juice

1 carrot, chopped

1 tsp chia seeds

1 tsp grated ginger

Directions:

Combine all ingredients in a blender, and blend until smooth. Enjoy!

Strawberry and Coconut Smoothie

Serves: 2

Prep time: 5 min

Ingredients:

3-4 ice cubes

1½ cup coconut milk

2 cups fresh strawberries

1 tsp chia seeds

Directions:

Place all ingredients in a blender and purée until smooth. Enjoy!

Beautiful Skin Smoothie

Serves: 2

Prep time: 5 min

Ingredients:

1 cup frozen strawberries

1½ cup green tea

1 peach, chopped

½ avocado

5-6 raw almonds

1 tsp coconut oil

Directions:

Place all ingredients in a blender and purée until smooth. Enjoy!

Kiwi and Pear Smoothie

Serves: 2

Prep time: 5 min

Ingredients:

1 frozen banana, chopped

3 oranges, juiced

2 kiwi, peeled and halved

1 pear, chopped

1 tbsp coconut butter

Directions:

Juice oranges and combine all ingredients in a blender then blend until smooth. Enjoy!

Tropical Smoothie

Serves: 2

Prep time: 5 min

Ingredients:

2-3 ice cubes

1½ cup coconut water

½ avocado

1 mango, peeled, diced

1 cup pineapple, chopped

2-3 dates, pitted

Directions:

Place all ingredients in a blender and purée until smooth. Enjoy!

Melon Smoothie

Serves: 2

Prep time: 5 min

Ingredients:

1 frozen banana, chopped

1-2 frozen broccoli florets

1 cup coconut water

½ honeydew melon, cut in pieces

1 tsp chia seeds

Directions:

Combine all ingredients in a blender, and blend until smooth.

Healthy Skin Smoothie

Serves: 2

Prep time: 5 min

Ingredients:

1 cup frozen berries

1 cup almond milk

½ avocado

1 pear

1 tbsp ground pumpkin seeds

1 tsp vanilla extract

Directions :

Put all ingredients in a blender and blend until smooth. Enjoy!

Paleo Dessert Smoothie

Serves: 2

Prep time: 5 min

Ingredients:

1 frozen banana

1 cup coconut water

1 cup raspberries

2 apricots, chopped

1 tbsp almond butter

Directions:

Put all ingredients into blender. Blend until smooth. Enjoy!

Easy Superfood Smoothie

Serves: 2

Prep time: 5 min

Ingredients:

3-4 ice cubes

1½ cup green tea

1 pear, chopped

½ cup blueberries

½ cup blackberries

1 tbsp almond butter

Directions :

Place all ingredients in a blender and blend for until even. Enjoy!

Antioxidant Smoothie

Serves: 2

Prep time: 5 min

Ingredients:

1 cup frozen raspberries

1½ cups orange juice

2 kiwi, peeled and halved

1 tsp chia seeds

1 tsp ground pumpkin seeds

Directions:

Blend all ingredients in a blender until smooth. Enjoy!

Coconut and Date Smoothie

Serves: 2

Prep time: 5 min

Ingredients:

1 frozen banana, chopped

1½ cup coconut milk

2 leaves kale

15 dates, pitted

Directions:

Combine all ingredients in a blender and blend until smooth. Enjoy!

Kiwi and Grapefruit Smoothie

Serves: 2

Prep time: 5 min

Ingredients:

3-4 ice cubes

1½ cup grapefruit juice

1 banana, chopped

2 kiwi, cut

1 tsp sunflower seeds

Directions:

Juice the grapefruit then combine with the ice, kiwi and banana. Add a teaspoon of sunflower seeds and blend until smooth. Enjoy!

Mango and Nectarine Smoothie

Serves: 2

Prep time: 5 min

Ingredients:

3-4 ice cubes

1 cup almond milk

1 mango, peeled, diced

3 nectarines, chopped

1 tbsp ground flaxseed

Directions:

Put all ingredients into blender. Blend until smooth. Enjoy!

Pineapple Smoothie

Serves: 2

Prep time: 5 min

Ingredients:

2-3 ice cubes

2-3 oranges, juiced

2 cups pineapple, chopped

1 carrot, chopped

1 tbsp ground pumpkin seeds

1 tsp grated ginger

Directions:

Juice the oranges then combine with ice, carrot and pineapple in a blender. Add the pumpkin seeds ginger and blend until smooth. Enjoy!

Easy Vitamin Smoothie

Serves: 2

Prep time: 5 min

Ingredients:

2-3 ice cubes

2 pink grapefruits, juiced

½ avocado

1 carrot, chopped

1 cup strawberries

3-4 dates, pitted

Directions:

Juice the grapefruit then combine with ice and other ingredients. Blend until smooth. Enjoy!

About the Author

Vesela lives in Bulgaria with her family of six (including the Jack Russell Terrier). Her passion is going green in everyday life and she loves to prepare homemade cosmetic and beauty products for all her family and friends.

Vesela has been publishing her cookbooks for over a year now. If you want to see other healthy family recipes that she has published, together with some natural beauty books, you can check out her Author Page on Amazon.

Made in the USA
Coppell, TX
11 December 2021

68118659R00049